ILEOSTOMY DIET FOR GASTRONOMIC FREEDOM

A Quick Healing Nutrient Guide

Indulge In Healthful And Tasty Choices For A Happy Life

DR. SOFIA SILAS

Table of Contents

CHAPTER ONE 4

  Introduction 4

  Understanding Ileostomy..........................5

  The Importance Of Diet Following Ileostomy Surgery...6

  Nutritional Needs After Ileostomy................7

CHAPTER TWO 10

  Navigating Food Options With An 10

  Developing A Balanced Ileostomy 12

  Foods To Include In Your..............................16

CHAPTER THREE..20

  Foods To Avoid With An Ileostomy..............20

  Tips For Cooking And Preparing...................23

  Managing Digestive Issues And...................26

CHAPTER FOUR 29

  Hydration And Fluid Intake For Patients With Ileostomy 29

  Exploring Supplements For 32

  Meal Planning Strategies For 36

CHAPTER FIVE 39

Eating Out And Socializing With An Ileostomy
....39

Travel Tips For Ileostomy Patients...............42

Physical Activity And Exercise 43

Accepting Dietary Changes For 45

Overcoming Challenges And 46

Conclusion..49

CHAPTER ONE

Introduction

Ileostomy surgery may be a life-changing operation for those suffering from inflammatory bowel disease (IBD), colorectal cancer, or other digestive issues. While it relieves symptoms and improves quality of life, it also causes major changes in food patterns.

Understanding how to handle food and nutrition after ileostomy surgery is critical for overall health and well-being. In this talk, we'll look at the notion of an ileostomy, the necessity of food thereafter, nutritional requirements, and ways for developing a balanced diet plan.

Understanding Ileostomy

An ileostomy is a surgical technique that includes making an incision in the belly and bringing a piece of the small intestine, known as the ileum, to the surface to establish a stoma. This stoma acts as an alternate route for waste removal when the usual route via the colon and rectum is not working properly.

Ileostomies may be temporary or permanent, depending on the underlying medical problem and the scope of surgical intervention necessary.

The Importance Of Diet Following Ileostomy Surgery

Following ileostomy surgery, patients must adjust to considerable changes in their digestive tract.

Because the colon and rectum are bypassed, the ileostomy produces liquid or semi-liquid feces, which may cause issues such as dehydration, electrolyte imbalances, and vitamin shortages if not controlled effectively. As a result, keeping a healthy diet becomes critical to supporting general health and avoiding issues.

Nutritional Needs After Ileostomy

Following ileostomy surgery, the body's capacity to absorb certain nutrients may be impaired. Factors such as lower intestinal surface area and quicker transit time might impact nutrient absorption, necessitating careful dietary choices. Key nutrients that may need particular care are:

1. Monitor and supplement electrolyte levels, especially sodium, potassium, and magnesium, to avoid shortages

and maintain appropriate body functioning.

2. Fluids: Staying hydrated is vital to avoid dehydration, particularly with the increased risk of fluid loss via stoma output. Consuming lots of water and electrolyte-rich drinks may help you stay hydrated.

3. Protein is required for tissue repair and maintenance, especially after surgery. Consuming high-quality protein sources such as lean meats, poultry, fish, eggs, dairy, legumes, and tofu may aid in healing and general health.

4. Vitamins and minerals: Post-ileostomy alterations in digestive function may influence vitamin B12, iron, calcium, and vitamin D levels. Working with a healthcare physician or nutritionist to ensure appropriate intake via food and supplements is critical.

CHAPTER TWO
Navigating Food Options With An Ileostomy

Adjusting to life with an ileostomy entails understanding how various meals affect stoma output and general digestive health. While no stringent dietary limits exist, some foods may be more prone to produce problems such as increased stool production, gas, or stink. Common triggers include:

1. High-fiber meals, such as fresh fruits and vegetables, whole grains, nuts, and seeds, might be difficult to digest and cause

blockages or excessive stoma output. Cooking or preparing certain meals may make them more palatable.

2. Gas-producing foods: Beans, cabbage, broccoli, onions, and carbonated drinks may cause gas and discomfort. Modifying consumption or choosing fewer gas-forming options might help alleviate symptoms.

3. Consuming spicy or acidic meals, such as citrus fruits, tomatoes, and vinegar, might irritate the digestive system, leading to increased stoma output and pain. It may be useful to

monitor individual tolerance levels and restrict intake of certain foods.

Developing A Balanced Ileostomy Diet Plan

Designing a healthy diet plan after ileostomy surgery entails including a range of nutrient-dense foods while keeping individual tolerances and preferences in mind. Some basic guidelines for developing a healthy ileostomy food plan include:

1. Eating modest, frequent meals may help regulate stoma output and reduce stomach pain.

2. Maintaining hydration: Drinking enough of fluids, such as water and electrolyte-rich drinks, is crucial for avoiding dehydration and staying hydrated, especially during hot weather or physical exercise.

3. Including protein-rich meals in every meal helps promote healing, muscular maintenance, and general wellness. Lean meats, poultry, fish, eggs, dairy, lentils, and tofu are all great alternatives.

4. Choose nutrient-dense foods: Consuming fruits, vegetables, whole grains, lean meats, and healthy fats may provide

nutritional demands without causing digestive difficulties.

5. Listen to your body. Understanding how various meals influence stoma output, energy levels, and general well-being may aid in identifying unique triggers and making educated dietary decisions.

To summarize, managing food and nutrition following ileostomy surgery is critical for preserving health, avoiding problems, and promoting general well-being. Understanding the particular problems and nutritional requirements connected with an ileostomy may assist people in developing a well-balanced meal plan that suits their specific needs and preferences. Working closely with healthcare specialists, especially dietitians, may give important advice and support throughout the postoperative period.

Living with an ileostomy has unique problems, especially in terms of food and nutrition. Whether you've just had ileostomy surgery or have been living with one for a long, knowing what foods to eat, what to avoid, and how to manage meals is critical for preserving your health and wellness.

Foods To Include In Your Ileostomy Diet

Maintaining a balanced and healthy diet is crucial for everyone, but it is especially important for those who have an ileostomy. Here are some meals that are typically well-tolerated and useful for people with ileostomies:

1. Choose lean proteins such as skinless chicken, fish, eggs, tofu, and lentils. These meals give the essential amino acids required for tissue repair and general wellness

without producing excessive stool production.

2. Soft fruits, such as bananas, avocados, peeled apples, and ripe melons, are soft on the digestive tract and reduce the risk of stoma obstructions or discomfort.

3. Cooked veggies (carrots, spinach, zucchini, and potatoes) are simpler to digest than raw ones. Steaming or cooking veggies until soft might help relieve intestinal pain.

4. White Grains: Choose refined grains like white rice, bread, and pasta prepared with white flour. These grains are less prone to

irritate or clog the digestive system than whole grains rich in fiber.

5. Consider dairy alternatives for lactose intolerant or sensitive individuals, such as lactose-free milk, almond milk, or soy milk. These options provide calcium and vitamin D without causing intestinal problems.

6. Smooth nut butter, such as almond or peanut butter, provides protein and healthful fats. However, they must be consumed in moderation, since too much fat might cause loose stools.

7. Probiotic Foods: Consuming probiotic-rich foods like yogurt,

kefir, sauerkraut, and kimchi help improve gut health and bowel motions. Probiotics promote a healthy balance of intestinal flora, lowering the risk of digestive issues.

CHAPTER THREE

Foods To Avoid With An Ileostomy

While many meals are safe for people who have an ileostomy, some may aggravate symptoms or create problems. The following foods should be avoided or consumed in moderation.

1. Fibrous meals, such as nuts, seeds, popcorn, raw vegetables, and whole grains, may be difficult to digest and produce stoma irritation or obstructions. Limit your consumption of these items or go for cooked and peeled variants.

2. Gas-Producing Foods: Beans, cabbage, broccoli, onions, and carbonated drinks may cause bloating and discomfort. Monitor your consumption of these items and try eating them in lesser quantities.

3. Spicy and acidic meals, including citrus fruits, tomatoes, and vinegar-based goods, might irritate the digestive system and create pain. These foods should be avoided or consumed in moderation, particularly if you suffer from acid reflux or inflammation.

4. High-fat meals: Consuming greasy or fried meals might increase bowel motions and cause loose stools or diarrhea. Limit your consumption of fatty meals such as fried meats, butter, cream sauces, and fast food to avoid stomach problems.

5. Excess sugar and artificial sweeteners may cause diarrhea and dehydration. Choose natural sweeteners sparingly and study food labels carefully.

6. Tough Meats: Fibrous meat products, such as jerky, may be difficult to chew and digest. To

ease digestion, use soft cuts of meat or other protein sources.

Tips For Cooking And Preparing Meals With An Ileostomy

Cooking and preparing meals with an ileostomy necessitates certain changes to guarantee proper digestion and comfort. Here are a few suggestions to make dinner easier:

1. Chew thoroughly. Take your time chewing food properly to help digestion and limit the possibility of blockages. Avoid taking huge pieces and eat slowly to help your

body metabolize food more efficiently.

2. Stay hydrated. Drink lots of fluids throughout the day to avoid dehydration, particularly if you have increased stool production. Aim for at least eight glasses of water each day and minimize caffeinated or sugary drinks.

3. Monitor portion sizes. Pay attention to portion amounts to avoid overeating, which may strain your digestive system. Eating smaller, more frequent meals throughout the day may aid digestion and reduce pain.

4. Experiment with cooking methods. Investigate alternative cooking techniques such as baking, steaming, or grilling to prepare meals that are simpler to digest. Avoid frying or charbroiling, which may increase fat and cause stomach difficulties.

5. Maintain a food diary to detect trigger foods or digestive habits. This knowledge may help you make more educated decisions and change your diet to properly manage symptoms.

Managing Digestive Issues And Nutritional Absorption

Despite cautious dietary choices, people with ileostomies may still have digestive problems or difficulty absorbing specific nutrients. Here are some approaches to addressing these concerns:

1. If your diet doesn't supply enough nutrients, see your healthcare professional about supplementation options. Vitamin B12, calcium, and iron are common supplements for people with ileostomies.

2. Consult with a Dietitian: A certified dietitian who specializes in gastrointestinal health may provide a specific dietary plan. A dietitian can help you optimize your food intake, manage digestive issues, and address particular dietary concerns.

3. Practice Mindful Eating. Be conscious of how you eat and pay attention to your body's signals. To avoid overeating or discomfort, avoid distractions when eating, chew your meal fully, and stop when you're full.

4. Seek Medical Advice: If you have chronic digestive concerns

including stomach discomfort, diarrhea, or bloating, see your doctor for examination and treatment. These symptoms might signal underlying digestive issues that need medical treatment.

By implementing these dietary suggestions and practical advice into your daily routine, you may properly manage your ileostomy while also enjoying a diverse and healthy diet that promotes your overall health and well-being. Remember to focus on balance, moderation, and listening to your body's demands to improve digestion and reduce any issues.

CHAPTER FOUR

Hydration And Fluid Intake For Patients With Ileostomy

Hydration is an important part of sustaining health and well-being for those with ileostomy. An ileostomy is a surgical operation that produces an incision in the belly through which the small intestine protrudes, diverting feces into a pouch worn outside the body.

This change in the digestive tract may affect fluid absorption and electrolyte balance, making it critical for ileostomy patients to monitor their hydration and fluid intake.

One of the most common concerns for ileostomy patients is the risk of dehydration. With a section of the small intestine bypassed, the body may have a diminished capacity to absorb water and electrolytes, increasing the risk of dehydration. As a result, maintaining appropriate fluid intake is critical to avoiding dehydration and its accompanying problems.

Ileostomy patients should consume lots of fluids throughout the day, preferably hydrating liquids such as water, herbal teas, and clear soups. To aid absorption and avoid overloading the digestive system, fluid consumption should be spaced out evenly throughout the day rather than consumed in excessive quantities all at once.

Electrolyte balance is another concern for ileostomy patients since the operation might impair the body's capacity to control electrolytes including sodium, potassium, and chloride. Including electrolyte-rich foods and drinks in your diet may help you maintain a healthy balance. Foods such as bananas, potatoes, coconut water, and sports drinks may help restore electrolytes lost during ileostomy output.

Ileostomy patients must monitor their urine production and be aware of indicators of dehydration such as dark urine, dry mouth, weariness, and dizziness. If you suspect dehydration, get medical assistance right once and, if required, get intravenous fluids to rehydrate.

Exploring Supplements For Ileostomy Patients

In addition to maintaining correct hydration and electrolyte balance, ileostomy patients may benefit from certain supplements that promote general health and well-being. However, it is critical to speak with a healthcare expert before beginning any new supplements, since individual requirements may differ depending on variables such as diet, medical history, and prescription use.

One significant worry among ileostomy patients is the possibility of nutritional shortages owing to alterations in digestion and absorption. Certain vitamins and minerals may be less readily absorbed following ileostomy surgery, necessitating supplementation for certain patients. Vitamin B12, calcium, vitamin D, and iron are some of the minerals that may need supplementation in specific circumstances.

Probiotics are another supplement that some ileostomy patients can find useful. Probiotics are living microorganisms that may improve gut health by fostering a healthy bacterial balance in the digestive system. This is especially essential for those with changed gut architecture, such as those who have an ileostomy, since it may help avoid complications like pouchitis and bacterial development.

Fiber supplements may also be beneficial for ileostomy patients, but it is important to approach with caution and contact a healthcare expert before incorporating fiber into the diet.

While some people may benefit from fiber supplements to thicken their stool and control their bowel movements, others may find that it worsens symptoms like gas, bloating, or intestinal blockage.

Meal Planning Strategies For Ileostomy Patients

Meal planning may help you manage your ileostomy while also preserving your general health and well-being. Individuals with an ileostomy may avoid dehydration, electrolyte imbalances, and digestive pain by carefully choosing foods and organizing meals.

When preparing meals for ileostomy patients, it is important to concentrate on foods that are readily digested and mild on the digestive tract. This may contain cooked fruits and vegetables, lean meats like chicken or fish, and whole grains that have been well-cooked or processed to a finer texture.

It is also critical for ileostomy patients to monitor their fiber intake and choose meals that are acceptable for their specific tolerance levels. While some people may handle high-fiber diets without problems, others may find that fiber aggravates symptoms like gas, bloating, or intestinal blockage. Experimenting with various fiber kinds and quantities might help you figure out what works best for you.

Another option for ileostomy patients is to consume smaller, more often meals throughout the day rather than larger ones.

This may assist in avoiding overloading the digestive system and may lower the likelihood of problems like pouch leakage or pain.

CHAPTER FIVE

Eating Out And Socializing With An Ileostomy

Individuals with an ileostomy have particular obstacles while eating out and socializing, but with good planning and preparation, it is perfectly feasible to enjoy dining experiences while efficiently managing the disease.

When eating out, it might be beneficial to do your homework ahead of time and find places that provide a diverse menu, including foods acceptable for those with dietary restrictions or digestive disorders. Many restaurants are happy to accommodate specific requests or dietary restrictions, so don't be afraid to convey your requirements to the waitstaff or chef.

It's also important to be cautious of meal sizes and avoid overeating since eating too much at once might raise the chance of digestive discomfort or pouch leakage. Consider ordering appetizers or small plates instead of entire dinners, or request a take-out container to keep leftovers for later.

When conversing with friends or family, communication is

essential. Do not be reluctant to talk about your dietary preferences or constraints with your companions; they may be more understanding and helpful than you anticipate. Bringing your snacks or meals to events may also assist ensure that you have alternatives that are safe and meet your dietary requirements.

Overall, with careful planning, attention to hydration and nutrition, and open communication with healthcare experts and loved ones, people with ileostomies may live productive and rewarding lives while efficiently managing their illness.

Travel Tips For Ileostomy Patients

Living with an ileostomy may provide unique problems, but it should not limit your ability to travel and enjoy the globe. With good planning and awareness, you may enjoy your trip while properly managing your health. Here is some crucial advice for ileostomy patients to make their vacation experience smoother and more pleasurable.

Physical Activity And Exercise Recommendations

Maintaining an active lifestyle is essential for general health and well-being, particularly for ileostomy patients. Regular exercise not only strengthens muscles and improves cardiovascular health, but it also helps with stress management and mood enhancement. However, it is essential to undertake physical exercise with prudence and care for your health.

Walking, swimming, cycling, and yoga are all low-impact activities that ileostomy patients handle well. These exercises boost fitness levels without placing too much pressure on the abdomen. To prevent overexertion, start small and gradually increase the intensity and length of your exercises.

When doing active activities, keep your stoma and ostomy equipment in mind. Wearing supportive clothes and an ostomy belt might assist in securing your pouch and keep it from moving or leaking when exercising. Stay hydrated and take pauses as required, paying attention to your body's cues to minimize exhaustion or pain.

Accepting Dietary Changes
For Gastronomic Freedom

Adjusting to dietary changes is an important part of life with an ileostomy. While certain foods should be avoided or taken in moderation to avoid difficulties like blockages or excessive output, it is still feasible to have a diverse and enjoyable diet.

Consuming high-fiber diets, lean meats, fruits, and vegetables may assist support good digestion and avoid stoma concerns. Chew your meal fully and drink lots of water throughout the day to help digestion and avoid dehydration.

When traveling, carefully organize your meals and snacks to ensure that you have access to appropriate selections that will not exacerbate your illness. Pack portable, readily digested snacks like granola bars, almonds, fruits, and crackers to have on hand when visiting new places.

Overcoming Challenges And Celebrating Success

Traveling with an ileostomy may bring some difficulties, but with careful preparation and an optimistic attitude, you may overcome barriers and have unforgettable experiences. Here are some frequent issues experienced by ileostomy patients when traveling and how to deal with them:

1. Check bathroom access at your location and bring supplies including wipes, ostomy pouches, and disposal bags for emergencies.

2. Inform airline workers or other transportation providers about your illness ahead of time to seek adjustments, such as priority boarding or aisle seats for easy lavatory access.

3. Pack additional ostomy supplies, such as pouches,

adhesives, and barrier rings, to prepare for unforeseen scenarios.

4. Managing changes in routine: Maintain your usual ostomy care routine, such as emptying and changing your pouch at regular intervals to avoid leaks and skin irritation.

Despite these limitations, traveling with an ileostomy may be very fulfilling and inspiring. Celebrate your accomplishments along the journey, whether they include navigating a new city, sampling new delicacies, or just spending quality time with loved ones. Remember that having an ileostomy does not define you or restrict your capacity to explore the world.

Conclusion

Traveling with an ileostomy requires careful preparation, adaptability, and a cheerful attitude. By following these guidelines and advice, you may have enjoyable and memorable vacation experiences while efficiently managing your health.

Accept dietary modifications, be physically active, and don't allow obstacles to prevent you from discovering new places and creating great experiences. With the proper preparation and mindset, you may travel confidently and enjoy all the world has to offer.